YOUR KNOWLEDGE HAS VALUE

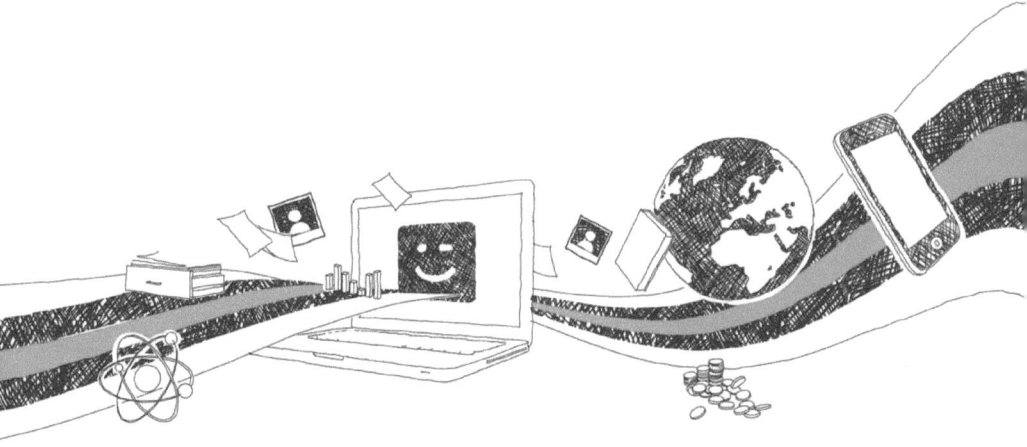

- We will publish your bachelor's and master's thesis, essays and papers

- Your own eBook and book - sold worldwide in all relevant shops

- Earn money with each sale

Upload your text at www.GRIN.com
and publish for free

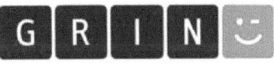

Bibliographic information published by the German National Library:

The German National Library lists this publication in the National Bibliography; detailed bibliographic data are available on the Internet at http://dnb.dnb.de .

This book is copyright material and must not be copied, reproduced, transferred, distributed, leased, licensed or publicly performed or used in any way except as specifically permitted in writing by the publishers, as allowed under the terms and conditions under which it was purchased or as strictly permitted by applicable copyright law. Any unauthorized distribution or use of this text may be a direct infringement of the author s and publisher s rights and those responsible may be liable in law accordingly.

Imprint:

Copyright © 2012 GRIN Verlag, Open Publishing GmbH
Print and binding: Books on Demand GmbH, Norderstedt Germany
ISBN: 9783668223424

This book at GRIN:

http://www.grin.com/en/e-book/321593/does-smoking-increase-the-risk-of-lumbar-disc-prolapse-in-individuals-aged

Shoab Ahmad

Does smoking increase the risk of lumbar disc prolapse in individuals aged from 20 to 40 years?

Smoking as a risk factor for disc prolapse

GRIN Publishing

GRIN - Your knowledge has value

Since its foundation in 1998, GRIN has specialized in publishing academic texts by students, college teachers and other academics as e-book and printed book. The website www.grin.com is an ideal platform for presenting term papers, final papers, scientific essays, dissertations and specialist books.

Visit us on the internet:

http://www.grin.com/

http://www.facebook.com/grincom

http://www.twitter.com/grin_com

Does smoking increase the risk of lumbar disc prolapse in individuals aged from 20 to 40 years?

A research protocol design

Shoab Ahmad

SCHOOL OF POPULATION HEALTH
FACULTY OF MEDICINE, DENTISTRY &
HEALTH SCIENCE
THE UNIVERSITY OF MELBOURNE

RESEARCH PROJECT IN
EPIDEMIOLOGY/BIOSTATISTICS
MASTERS OF PUBLIC HEALTH
(POPH90219)

JUNE 8, 2012

Disclaimer

The work in this research report was undertaken for the requirement of The University of Melbourne for the degree of Master of Public Health. The views expressed are those of the author and may not reflect the view of The University of Melbourne, School of Population Health.

Acknowledgements

I would like to show my sincere gratitude to my supervisor and mentor Dr. Gillian

Dite, for acting as a sounding board as I developed this research protocol. Thanks for

you guidance and encouragement.

I would also like to express my gratitude to Assoc. Prof. Mark Jenkins, subject

coordinator for his supervision and advice in conducting this project.

Abstract

Introduction

Lumbar disc prolapse is one of the most common neurological conditions and there has been no agreement on its appropriate management. Lumbar disc prolapse is a very common cause of a clinical spectrum of symptoms including back pain, sciatica, knee pain and numbness, and in severe cases, nerve damage and loss of bladder and bowel control. Back pain is the most common symptom of lumbar disc prolapse and is one of the most common conditions for which a patient seeks medical attention. The primary aim of this research project is to design a protocol that estimates the effect of smoking on the risk of lumbar disc prolapse in individuals aged from 20 to 40 years.

Background

Evidence suggests that smokers have a 3-4 times higher risk of developing disc disease and that smoking can exacerbate pre-existing disc degeneration. Nicotine and other harmful toxins in cigarette smoke prevent nucleosus pulposus and annulus fibrosus cells from up taking nutrients. This can cause significant inhibition of cell proliferation and extra cellular matrix synthesis, making disc injury more likely and recovery from an injury slow. While there is strong evidence in the literature that smoking does have a role in the pathogenesis of lumbar disc prolapse and back pain, there are no accurate estimates of the magnitude of the increased risk.

Methods

Different analytical study designs were evaluated to assess their strengths, limitations and feasibility for answering the research question. Issues of subject selection, bias and measurement were assessed for case-control and cohort study designs. It was concluded that the most epidemiologically robust design would be a case-control study, which was chosen for its efficiency in time and cost.

Results

Cases will be chosen from orthopaedic, neurological and physiotherapy wards from hospitals across Australia and controls will be chosen from neighbourhood of the cases. The primary outcome will be lumbar disc prolapse confirmed on either computerised tomography (CT) scan or magnetic resonance imaging (MRI). Exposure assessment will be conducted during a face-to-face interview by trained interviewers using a structured questionnaire, to minimise bias. Statistical analysis will be conducted using Stata 11, using logistic regression techniques and adjusting for potential confounders.

Discussion

Considering the relative rarity of lumbar disc prolapse and number of true cases, the study has to be conducted all across Australian hospitals to recruit the high number of cases required for the study to have sufficient power to detect an odds ratio of 1.5. Controls could have been recruited from the same hospitals but might have introduced selection bias.

Conclusion

A case-control study is the best design to realise the primary aim of this research protocol. Conducting the study across Australia will enable enough cases to be identified and recruiting controls from the neighborhood of the cases with simple enrolment requirements will increase the response rate and minimise the bias. Exposure measurement through face-to-face interview by trained interviewers using a structured questionnaire is cost efficient, and the use of trained interviewers ensures that participants understand the questions clearly.

Table of Contents

Table of Figures

1. Introduction

Lumbar disc prolapse is one of the most common neurological conditions (Broetz,

Hahn et al. 2008) and has a vast spectrum of symptoms including back pain, pain and

numbness around the knees, sciatica, severe nerve damage and loss of bladder and

bowel control (Heliovaara, Impivaara et al. 1987) (Weber 1994). These symptoms can

cause severe disability, and back pain as a result of lumbar disc prolapse is one of the

most common conditions for which a patient seeks medical attention (Manek and

MacGregor 2005). There is little agreement on the appropriate management of lumbar

disc prolapse (Broetz, Hahn et al. 2008).

The known risk factors for lumbar disc prolapse include age, sex, high body mass

index (BMI), and occupations such as night shift workers, athletes, drivers and heavy

weight lifters. Some studies have shown that smoking is associated with a higher

incidence of lumbar disc prolapse (Akmal, Kesani et al. 2004). *In-vitro* studies of

non-human spinal disc showed that smoking does have detrimental effect on

nucleolus pulposus cells (Akmal, Kesani et al. 2004). Recent studies have shown that

there is a genetic component to the risk of lumbar disc prolapse and back pain (Manek

and MacGregor 2005).

The widely accepted explanation for the effect of smoking on spinal disc cells is that

the nutritional uptake by disc cells is hampered by carboxy-hemoglobin present in the

blood of smokers (Gullihorn, Karpman et al. 2005), vasoconstriction (Miller, Clouse

et al. 2000) and changes in blood flow (Ernst 1993).

Of the general population, 60% to 80% experience back pain during their lifetime

(Riihimaki 1991). Lumbar disc prolapse and associated back pain pose huge

economic and public health burden (Hootman, Helmick et al. 2003). In Finland in

1980, around 3.7% of disability pensions granted to people aged from 30 to 64 years was due to lumbar disc prolapse, and 6% of work place disability could be attributed

to lumbar disc prolapses (Heliovaara, Impivaara et al. 1987). In people with lumbar

disc prolapse, the ability to perform routine daily work has been shown to be slightly

limited in 56%, at least markedly limited in 21% and severely limited in 5%

(Heliovaara, Impivaara et al. 1987). Additionally, around 51% of patients with lumbar

disc prolapse need long-term medical care including more than 10 visits to physicians,

hospitals, surgical or neurosurgical specialists within 12 months (Heliovaara,

Impivaara et al. 1987). This recurrent use of medical assistance was specifically

common in patients with lumbar disc prolapse, and 5% was directly attributed to

lumbar disc prolapse related back pain (Heliovaara, Impivaara et al. 1987).

2. Background

2.1 Disease overview

Lumbar disc prolapse occurs when the soft gelatinous nucleus pulposus of vertebral

disc extrudes though weakened walls of the annulus fibrosus resulting in compression

of the adjacent nerve roots (Figure 1) (Heliovaara, Impivaara et al. 1987). The

association between the extent of lumbar disc prolapse and clinical signs and

symptoms is not properly understood (Masui, Yukawa et al. 2005) (Komori, Okawa et

al. 1998) but common symptoms due to compression of nerve roots range from back

pain, knee pain, numbness around the knees, sciatica to loss of bladder and bowel

control in cases of severe spinal cord compression (Heliovaara, Impivaara et al. 1987)

(Weber 1994).

Figure 1 Diagrammatic representation of prolapsed disc and compression of

nerve root *

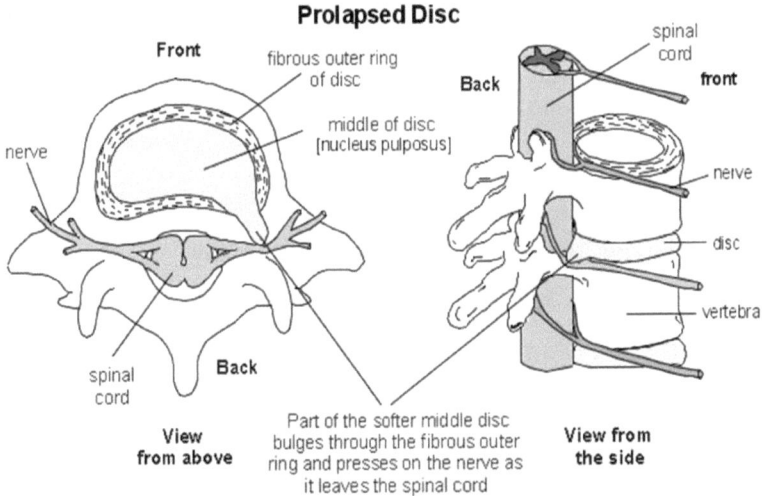

*Image source: http://www.patient.co.uk/pdf/pilsL762.pdf#

In Australia, in 1998, back problems affected 5.4% of the total population, making it one of the most common musculoskeletal conditions following arthritis (AIHW 2006). In 1995, the National Health Survey of Australia estimated the disease burden due to musculoskeletal conditions of the back to be 2,065 years lived with disability (YLD) for males and 1,903 YLD for females, and the overall incidence of back problems to be 65,938 per 100,000 individuals (Mathers, Vos et al. 2001). The 1995 National Health Survey also showed that around 2.2% of the population self-reported disorders of vertebral disc (Mathers, Vos et al. 2001). These estimates may be unreliable as they were calculated from self-reported data and therefore the accurate estimates of incidence and prevalence of lumbar disc prolapse are not available.

2.2 Anatomy of spinal disc

The intervertebral disc is a fibro-cartilagenous structure enclosed between hyaline cartilagenous end plates of the adjacent vertebral bodies (Figure 2) (Cassinelli and Kang 2000).

Figure 2 Diagrammatic coronal views of vertebral bodies and disc*

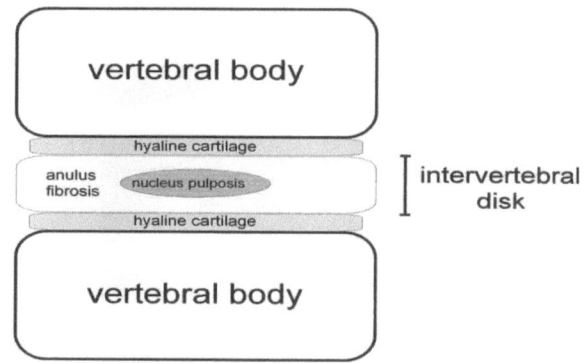

*Image source:

http://www.iupui.edu/~anatd502/Labs.f04/cartilage%20&%20bone%20lab/Bone%20&%20Cartilage%20%20Lab.html

The intervertebral disc is composed of concentrically arranged tissue layers

(Cassinelli and Kang 2000). The outer part is the annulus fibrosus and is made of

dense, highly oriented collagen lamellae and the inner part is soft gelatinous nucleus

pulposus (Figure 3) (Cassinelli and Kang 2000).

Figure 3 Diagrammatic sagittal view of a vertebral disc

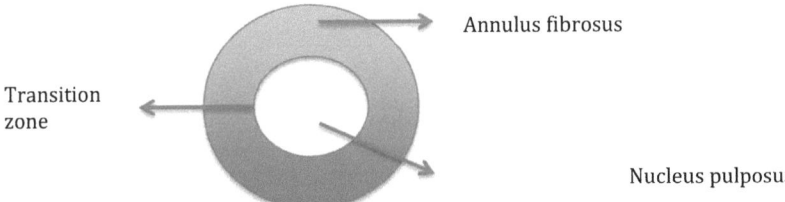

Annulus fibrosus

Transition
zone

Nucleus pulposus

Outer annulus fibrosus and centrally located gelatinous nucleus pulposus are

separated by a thin fibrous tissue called as the transition zone (Trout, Buckwalter et

al. 1982).

Intervertebral discs have limited vessel innervations and are relatively hypo-vascular

(Cassinelli and Kang 2000). The primary mechanism for the nutrition of the inner disc

is through diffusion of nutrients and metabolites across the end plates of their adjacent

vertebral bodies (Cassinelli and Kang 2000). Inner regions of the disc are without

innervations as free nerve endings penetrate only a short distance into the annulus

fibrosus (Jackson, Winkelmann et al. 1966) (Ashton, Ashton et al. 1992).

Special arrangement of the collagen in the outer layers of annulus fibrosus provide

tensile strength of the intervertebral disc, stability between vertebrae and prevents

bulging of disc in response to load (Ostrum, Romy et al. 1993).

2.3 Diagnosis of lumbar disc prolapse

The usual presenting complaint to a physician is back pain, which can be

accompanied by pain radiating along the buttock to the back of one or both legs and numbness around the knees (Heliovaara, Impivaara et al. 1987). In severe cases of

lumbar disc prolapse, the patient can present with a loss of bladder and bowel control,

due to nerve root compression (Weber 1994). The diagnosis is usually made on

clinical history and examination, but can only be confirmed only through

computerised tomography (CT) or Magnetic resonance imaging (MRI) (Figures 4 &

5) (Deyo, Loeser et al. 1990).

Figure 4 Magnetic resonance image (MRI) of lumbar disc prolapse (transverse
and sagittal views) *

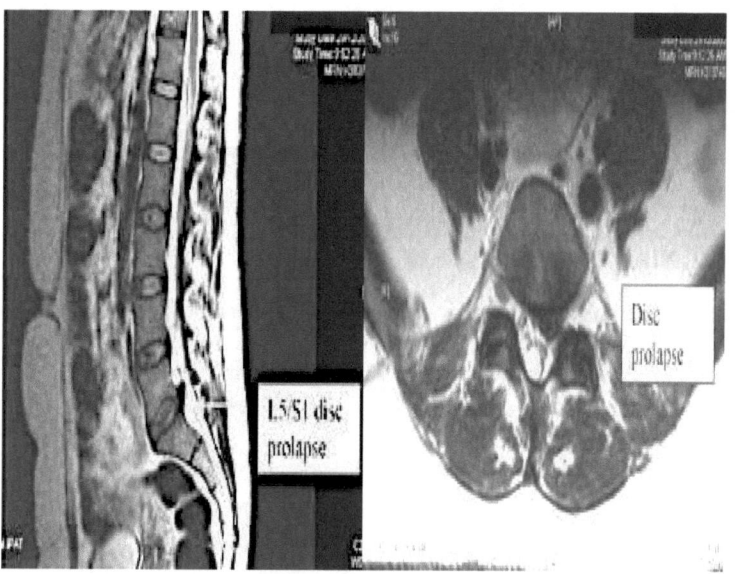

*Image source: http://www.vbsc.org.au/lumb_prolapse.htm

2.4 Management

The usual management of lumbar disc prolapse is complete bed rest for few weeks,

analgesics, skeletal muscle relaxants and mechanical traction (Deyo, Loeser et al.

1990). It is known that the prolapsed portion of disc tends to decrease in size with

time (Bush, Cowan et al. 1992) which can be confirmed by MRI (Broetz, Hahn et al.

2008). Physiotherapy and exercises to strengthen back muscles are advised to prevent

relapses (Broetz, Hahn et al. 2008). In severe cases of nerve compression or

compromised bladder or bowel control, immediate surgery is required to release

compression on the spinal cord (Deyo, Loeser et al. 1990).

2.5 Risk factors for lumbar disc prolapse

2.5.1 Age

Disc degeneration is a normal ageing process and usually begins in the second decade

of life (Powell, Szypryt et al. 1986). Disc degeneration is a common occurrence in the

second and third decades of life, and this degeneration of annulus fibrosus and

nucleus pulposus can reduce disc strength, making nucleus pulposus more likely to

prolapse (Powell, Szypryt et al. 1986).

One study demonstrated that the prevalence of degenerative disc disease increases

progressively with age from 6% under 20 years to 79% over 60 years, with over one

third aged 21 to 40 years showing abnormal disc on MRI (Powell, Szypryt et al.

1986). The same study found that 60% of subjects aged less than 40 years had some

degree of lumbar disc prolapse (Powell, Szypryt et al. 1986).

Another study found the mean age at the diagnosis of lumbar disc prolapse to be 40

years (Seidler, Bolm-Audorff et al. 2003). Another study of adolescents and young

adults found the prevalence of back pain to be 7% in subjects aged 12 to 22 years, and

suggested that there is a strong statistical association between back pain and age

(Hestbaek, Leboeuf-Yde et al. 2004). One study found that there was decline in

hospitalisations due to lumbar disc prolapse after the age of 49 years (Heliovaara,

Knekt et al. 1987).

The widely accepted explanation for lumbar disc prolapse becoming less common in older age is that there is a change in the consistency of the nucleus pulposus with advancing age (Ostrum, Romy et al. 1993). It becomes less gelatinous and more fibrous and there is nothing to bulge out (Ostrum, Romy et al. 1993).

2.5.2 Sex

Many studies have shown that the risk and prevalence of lumbar disc prolapse is higher for males. In one study conducted in Finland, the prevalence of lumbar disc prolapse was found to be higher in men 5.1% compared with women 3.7% (p<0.005) (Heliovaara, Impivaara et al. 1987). Another study found that men had a 1.6 times higher chance of lumbar disc prolapse than women (Heliovaara, Knekt et al. 1987).

2.5.3 High body mass index

Being overweight (body mass index (BMI) >= 25 kg/m^2) is strongly associated with an increased risk of disc degeneration and detrimental effects on the nucleus pulposus, changes which can be seen on MRI (adjusted odds ratio (OR) = 4.3, 95% confidence interval (95% CI) 1.3-14.3) and being overweight at young age (risk ratio (RR) 3.8, 95 % CI 1.4-10.4) was more strongly associated with disc degeneration than being overweight in middle age (RR 1.3, 95 % CI 0.7-2.7) (Liuke, Solovieva et al. 2005).

.2.5.4 Physical workload

There is a strong statistical association between lumbar disc prolapse and physical workload in the form of extreme forward bending, weight lifting or carrying heavy objects (Seidler, Bolm-Audorff et al. 2003). Another study has shown that there is an increased frequency of lumbar disc prolapse in foundry workers as compared to general population (Lawrence, Molyneux et al. 1966). Heavy lifting at work by agriculturalists, bricklayers, road menders, welders and heavy work done by miners, blacksmiths, carpenters and dock workers has also been shown to be associated with a higher incidence of lumbar disc prolapse (Braun 1969).

It has been found that there is increased risk of lumbar disc prolapse and hospitalisation in occupations requiring heavy physical workload such as wood, metal and construction workers (Heliovaara 1987). A case-control study showed that metal workers, construction workers who held their jobs for than 10 years had higher incidence of lumbar disc prolapse (Hofmann, Bolm-Audorff et al. 1997). Another case-control study has shown an increased incidence of lumbar disc prolapse in people lifting objects weighing more than 11.3 kg more than 25 times per day (Kelsey 1975).

2.5.5 Smoking

In an experimental study on rabbits, where 5000ng/kg nicotine was injected daily to two groups of 6 rabbits, for 4 weeks in the first group and 8 weeks in the second group, there were marked histological changes in spinal disc structures, such as the presence of spaces within the nucleus pulposus and separation from the adjacent annulus fibrosus (Afifi and Hafez 2007). The study also showed a dose-dependent relationship of these changes with amount of nicotine; "disc degeneration was more marked in rabbits injected with nicotine for 8 weeks than in those injected for 4 weeks" (Afifi and Hafez 2007). Nicotine has also been demonstrated to cause adverse morphologic changes in chick vertebral chondrocytes (Khan, Provenza et al. 1981), delayed bone healing (Hollinger, Schmitt et al. 1999) and higher failure rates of spinal vertebral fusion (Silcox III, Boden et al. 1998).

Many retrospective and prospective studies have shown that smokers do have higher incidence of back conditions (Ernst 1993). It has also been shown that back problems are positively associated with smoking history and number of packs smoked (Frymoyer, Pope et al. 1983). Another study has shown that, compared to non-smokers, the age and sex-adjusted OR for back symptoms increased in order for non-smokers, ex-smokers, pipe or cigar smokers and current smokers (Heliovaara, Makela et al. 1991).

Other effects of smoking and nicotine have been proposed as mediators of malnutrition in the intervertebral disc and include vasoconstriction (Miller, Clouse et al. 2000) and changes in blood flow (Ernst 1993).

In addition to nicotine, smoking introduces **carbon monoxide** into the blood stream. Carbon monoxide can inhibit absorption of nutrients from blood by the vertebral discs, making them dehydrated and less elastic (Holm and Nachemson 1988). "The discs can become malnourished and there is a greater risk of lumbar disc prolapse" (Holm and Nachemson 1988). Carbon monoxide can also interfere with the absorption of calcium which can lead to a weak vertebral structure (Holm and Nachemson 1988).

Other factor that indirectly associates lumbar disc prolapse and smoking is cough. Constant coughing is more prevalent among smokers due to chronic bronchitis, and can add to the risk of lumbar disc prolapse (Kelsey, Githens et al. 1984). During coughing, intra-abdominal pressure is increased, which in turn causes increased intradiscal pressure (Nachemson 1979) and repeated stress between discs (Kelsey, Githens et al. 1984). This puts added strain on the spine and discs, creating greater risk of lumbar disc prolapse (Kelsey, Githens et al. 1984).

2.5.6 Genetic factors

A study found that found that, when compared to dizygotic twins, monozygotic twins were more likely to report back pain if their co-twin also reported pain (Bengtsson and Thorson 1991). Another study showed a genetic association between sex and back pain as the self-reported back pain was higher in male twins than female twins (Jan Hartvigsen, Christensen et al. 2004). The same study suggested that "genetic factors are responsible for difference in the incidence of back pain in older men but there was no differences in older women" (Jan Hartvigsen, Christensen et al. 2004).

2.6 Summary

While there is strong evidence in the literature that smoking does have a role in the pathogenesis of lumbar disc prolapse and back pain, there is no accurate estimate of the magnitude of the increased risk (Mathers, Vos et al. 2001). Considering the implications of lumbar disc prolapse and its symptoms, not only for the patient but also for the whole healthcare infrastructure in terms of both tangible and intangible losses, there is urgent need for new research which would come up with true estimates of risk. This will aid in better understanding of the aetiology and epidemiology of lumbar disc prolapse, future research and will help in generation of new health promotion programs.

3. Issues for selecting study design

To answer the research question, an analytical study design is required to be able

estimate the association between smoking and lumbar disc prolapse. Considering the

nature of the proposed research question, descriptive studies, such as cross-sectional

and ecological study designs can be omitted because they cannot give an estimate of

association and can only give the incidence and prevalence of smoking and lumbar

disc prolapse. The analytical study designs that were evaluated were:

1. Randomised/non-randomised controlled trial (RCT/non-RCT).

2. Cohort (prospective and retrospective) study.

3. Case-control study.

3.1 Randomised/Non-Randomised controlled trial

➢ Strengths of RCT/non-RCT study.

By assigning the exposure in form of an intervention to one group and a placebo to

the other group, investigators can manipulate exposure. Temporality can be

established because exposure is given before the outcome is measured. It also helps in

the efficient investigation of the intervention as it allows exposure to be assigned, not

measured. It can provide strong evidence of causation as exposure is given first in

form of intervention and the outcome is measured later.

➢ Limitations of RCT/non-RCT study design

Issues with RCT/non-RCT study designs include problems with compliance and

cross-contamination where some people might not take the intervention assigned to

them and may seek alternative treatment. Then there are the issues of improper

randomisation, blinding and loss to follow-up, which can be high.

In this project, it is highly unethical and unfeasible to perform an RCT/non-RCT

because the exposure, smoking, is known to be extremely harmful - we cannot ethically ask people to take up smoking for research. Therefore an RCT/non-RCT study design cannot be chosen to answer the research question.

3.2 Cohort study design (prospective/retrospective)

➢ Strengths of cohort study design

o Prospective

Exposure and other risk factors data can be recorded precisely and temporality can be established as the cohort is initially disease free and is followed up over time. It can eliminate issue of recall bias. It is good for rare exposures but smoking is quite a common exposure. Multiple outcomes can be studied but the research question demands only one outcome. Incidence rate and risk can be calculated, which is the primary aim.

o Retrospective

It is cheaper and less time consuming than prospective cohort study. It is also useful for diseases that have long induction time or disease for which aetiology is not fully understood.

➢ Limitations of cohort study

o Prospective

The aetiology of lumbar disc prolapse is not fully understood and has long and unpredictable induction time. Therefore, conducting a prospective cohort study would be expensive and time-consuming. There is also the issue of reverse causation where some people might stop smoking if they are diagnosed with lumbar disc prolapse. Another major issue is loss to follow up.

o Retrospective

Lumbar disc prolapse is a rare disease and this can lead to limited control over choice

of cohort. Additionally, it may not be possible to identify the entire cohort, as there

are many asymptomatic cases of lumbar disc prolapse. The classification of exposure

is often crude and limited information on potential confounders can be obtained.

Although a prospective cohort study seems feasible to answer the research question,

because the pathogenesis and aetiology of lumbar disc prolapse is not fully

understood and it has a long and unpredictable induction time, it can be very time-

consuming and expensive. It therefore cannot be chosen as a study design to answer

the research question.

3.3 Case-control study design

➢ Strengths of case-control study

Case-control study is cheaper and less time-consuming compared with other study

designs. Measure of association in the form of an OR for exposure can be calculated.

Another advantage is that other risk factors and potential confounders can be included

in the analysis. It is generally good for rare outcomes and lumbar disc prolapse is a

rare outcome. It is also good when the study sample size is small, which is likely

given the rarity of lumbar disc prolapse. Therese is no issue of loss to follow up as

exposure and outcome data is measured at the same time.

➢ Limitations of case-control study

Bias can be introduced in the selection of both cases and controls and possible bias in

subjects agreeing to participate. Bias can be introduced in measurement as well. It is

generally not suitable for rare exposures but smoking is quite common. Case-control

studies cannot measure incidence risk or rate, but ORs can be estimated as a measure

of association. Case-control studies can be problematic in establishing the temporality of events, but in this study, it is unlikely that the timing of smoking history will be inaccurately recorded.

The case control study design seems best to answer the proposed research question, considering it is cheap and less time consuming, no issue of loss to follow-up, the relative rarity of lumbar disc prolapse and potential for examining other risk factors.

4. Issues to be considered for a case-control study

4.1 Identifying appropriate study population

Appropriate subjects for the proposed case-control study design can be identified using the principles outlined by (Elwood 2007).

4.1.1 Target population

The target population, to which result can be generalised, is all Australian people aged from 20 to 40 years and in other similar countries.

4.1.2 Source population

The source population, from which eligible subjects will be identified, is orthopaedic, neurosurgical and physiotherapy wards of hospitals across Australia. Subjects will be aged from 20 to 40 years.

4.1.3 Eligible population

Eligible population, from which study subjects can be chosen, will include:

Inclusion criteria/case definition

As the diagnosis of lumbar disc prolapse is made through clinical findings and confirmed through either CT or MRI. The true cases will be recent patients of lumbar disc prolapse aged between 20 to 40 years, which have been confirmed through, either of imaging technologies.

Exclusion criteria

Subjects who have had other spinal conditions such as back pain, osteochondrosis, spondylosis, scoliosis of spine, back injuries following trauma, malignancies of the spine, poliomyelitis and family history of any back condition.

Selection of cases

Cases meeting inclusion criteria can be recruited from orthopaedic, neurosurgical and physiotherapy departments from hospitals across Australia.

Selection of controls

Controls selected from hospitals will not necessarily represent the general population because they are at hospital- they are unwell. Therefore, controls will be recruited from the neighbourhood of the cases assuming that these neighbours will attend the same hospital and would therefore be a case if they developed lumbar disc prolapse. Neighbourhood controls have same exposure distribution, which is identical to distribution of the exposure in the cases (Grimes and Schulz 2005).

4.1.4 Study entrants

Study entrants include all eligible cases and controls from which written consent and requirement of enrolment can be taken.

4.1.5 Study participants

This includes all study entrants from which data can be collected for analysis.

4.2 Study sample size

Power based sample size calculation for a difference of two proportions, under assumptions:

1. Primary exposure of interest: Smoking.

2. Primary outcome of interest: Lumbar disc prolapse

3. Estimated prevalence of smoking in control group: 15% (Scollo, Winstanley et al. 2008).

4. Minimum clinically significant odds ratio (OR): 1.5

5. Ratio of cases and controls: 1:4

6. Significance (alpha): 0.05

7. Power (1- β): 0.8

Sample size calculation for a difference of two proportions in Stata 11 using:

Sampsi P_1 P_2, power (0.8) alpha (0.05) ratio (4)

Where $P_1 = P_{cases} = P2\ (OR) \div [1 + P2\ (OR - 1)]$

(Formula given in Stata 11 manual)

And $P_2 = P_{controls} = 0.15$

Therefore $P_1 = 0.209$, calculated using Microsoft Excel.

The estimated required sample size is 422 cases and 1688 controls. To allow for confounding by two variables, sex and occupation, the sample size can be increased by around 35% per group (Kirkwood and Stern 2003). No changes have been made in sample size for accounting loss to follow up, assuming it to be minimal.

The calculated sample size seems feasible to recruit, considering the study will be conducted across Australia.

4.3 Data collection

Data will be collected in detail for all the possible exposure variables: age, sex, weight, height, BMI, relevant personal history, occupation (type, physical workload, number of hours, day/night shift), relevant family history and smoking.

Data will be collected on a paper-based structured questionnaire (given in next section) by a trained interviewer at hospital or participant's home.

4.4 Sample questionnaire

A. Interviewer information

1. Interviewer ID

2. Form ID

3. Date of interview

4. Length of interview

5. Where was the interview conducted

   - Face-to-face at the respondents home/hospital

   - Face-to-face at another place (specify)

B. Background information: - Responder ID:

1. Age

2. Sex

3. Date of birth

4. Address (Post code only)

5. Marital status

6. Country of birth

7. Number of siblings

8. Weight

9. Height

10. Waist circumference

11. Body mass index

12. Occupation

13. Type of occupation (including length of shifts/day/night)

14. Number of years in current occupation

15. Previous occupation/s

16. Number of years in previous occupation/s

17. Highest level of education

C. Medical and surgical history

1. Any significant medical or surgical diagnosis or treatment

2. Any history of trauma

3. History of any fracture

4. History of polio vaccination

5. Any significant medical or surgical diagnosis or treatment for other family members

6. Any history of spinal trauma or malignancy

7. History of any visit to specialist

8. History of back pain (onset and duration)

9. History of any medication for back pain

10. History of any visit to physiotherapist

D. Smoking*

1. Do you smoke, if yes then what was your age when you first smoked?

2. Have you ever smoked a cigarette a day for 3 months or longer?

3. At what age did you first start smoking at least one cigarette per day for 3 months or longer?

4. During periods when you smoked regularly, on average how many cigarettes did you typically smoke in a day?

5. About two years ago were you smoking at least one cigarette a day?

6. Do you currently smoke at least one cigarette a day?

7. When did you last quit smoking regularly? (One cigarette a day for 3 months or longer)

8. How many years in total did you smoke at least one cigarette per day for 3 months or longer? (If you have stopped and restarted at least once, count only the time when you were smoking)

9. Have you ever smoked at least one cigar or one pipe per month for at least 3 months?

10. Did you smoke cigars/pipes or used other forms of smoking?

* Based on questionnaire available from

https://bioinformatics.dartmouth.edu/ccfrc/Downloads/RFQ.pdf

4.5 Potential sources of bias

4.5.1 Inappropriate selection of cases

Selection bias can be introduced into the study if selection of cases is not independent of their exposure status. This will possibly tend to bias the results away from the null hypothesis of no association between smoking and lumbar disc prolapse.

4.5.2 Inappropriate selection of controls

It is also possible that the eligible population might include some asymptomatic cases of lumbar disc prolapse, and for whom no confirmatory diagnosis has been made. This will possibly tend to bias the results towards the null hypothesis of no association between smoking and lumbar disc prolapse. Selection bias can also be introduced if controls are not selected independently of their exposure status i.e. if controls are selected based on their smoking status.

4.5.3 Differential participation rates

It is known that response, consent and enrolment rates among control subjects are usually low as compared to cases, which can lead to bias in the study. To avoid this, entrance requirements for control subjects can be kept simple and low so as to increase their participation. Response rates will be presented in the final analysis.

4.5.4 Differential errors in measuring exposure

Recall bias is the term used for differential measurement error in context of case-control studies. Cases generally tend to have good memory recall due to their awareness of their disease. Controls, on the other hand, generally tend to forget events, which are not related to any disease.

4.5.5 Non-differential errors in measurement

Non-differential error in measurement can introduce bias as well due to improperly designed questionnaire. This non-differential error will tend to bias the results towards the null hypothesis of no association between smoking and lumbar disc prolapse.

4.6 Potential confounders

To identify confounder, a causal model can be established and used.

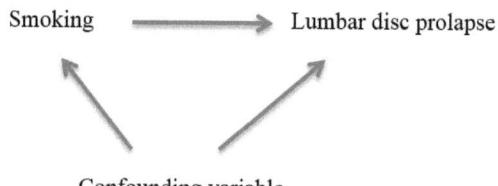

Research project Epidemiology/Biostatistics POPH90219

For a factor to be a confounder it has to meet the three conditions of being a

confounder (Rothman, Greenland et al. 2008):

1) Be associated with the outcome variable.

2) Be associated with the exposure variable.

3) Does not lie on the causal pathway between exposure and outcome.

Two important potential sources of confounding can be identified in the study, sex

and occupation.

➢ Sex can be a potential confounder as there is a strong association between sex and

smoking, males have higher rates of smoking as compared to females (Scollo,

Winstanley et al. 2008). It is also known that there is a strong association between sex

and lumbar disc prolapse, males have higher rates of lumbar disc prolapse as

compared to females (Heliovaara, Impivaara et al. 1987). Further it can be identified

that it in fact does not lie on the causal pathway and therefore can act as a confounder.

➢ Certain occupations have been linked to higher rates of smoking. "In the year 2004

smoking prevalence was higher (35%) in blue collar employment as compared to 14%

in white collar workers" (Scollo, Winstanley et al. 2008). It is known that there is

increased incidence of lumbar disc prolapse in certain occupations, requiring heavy

lifting and physical workload such as wood, metal and construction workers,

agriculturalists, bricklayers, road menders and welders (Seidler, Bolm-Audorff et al.

2003) (Pope, Magnusson et al. 1998) (Braun 1969) (Heliovaara 1987) (Hofmann,

Bolm-Audorff et al. 1997) (Kelsey 1975). Therefore occupation seems to be a

confounder as it is associated with exposure (smoking) and outcome (lumbar disc

prolapse) and does not seem lie on the causal pathway.

5. Statistical analysis

Analysis will be done using Stata 11. Histograms will be made for all the variables to check their distribution. Any outliers can be crosschecked with the original questionnaire to check for coding or data entry errors. Response and enrolment rates (number and percentage) will be reported for both case and control group as the number eligible, responded, enrolled and completed.

> ➤ **Univariate logistic regression**

Numbers and percentages for exposure variables by case and control status will be presented in tables. An overall (crude) exposure OR will be calculated using simple logistic regression. The likelihood ratio test will be used to test the null hypothesis of no association between smoking and lumbar disc prolapse.

	Outcome		Total
Exposure	Cases (Lumbar disc prolapse)	Controls (No lumbar disc prolapse)	
Smoker	A	B	A + B
Non-smoker	C	D	C + D
Total	A + C	B +D	A + B + C +D

Crude odds ratio (OR) (for unmatched case-control studies) = odds that cases were exposed/odds that controls were exposed (Webb and Bain 2011).

Odds that cases were exposed = A/C and odds that controls were exposed = B/D

Therefore the crude odds ratio (OR) = AxD/BxC

➤ Multiple logistic regression

Being an unmatched case-control design, unconditional multiple logistic regression
will be used to estimate ORs for the association between lumbar disc prolapse and
smoking. Model comparison will be made for risk factors and two potential
confounders, sex and occupation, to construct a final model, after adjusting for:

1. Sex and occupation: potential confounders.

2. Variables associated with smoking and lumbar disc prolapse after adjusting for sex.

3. Variables associated with smoking and lumbar disc prolapse after adjusting for
occupation.

4. Variables associated with lumbar disc prolapse after adjusting for sex.

5. Variables associated with lumbar disc prolapse after adjusting for occupation.

Evidence against the null hypothesis of no association between smoking and lumbar
disc prolapse will be assessed using likelihood ratio test.

6. Ethical issues

> **Ethics approval**

- Institutional review board, education department, hospitals and administrative authorities.

> **Informed consent**

- Consent will be sought prior to the study by providing plain language statement to the participants.

> **Harms and benefits**

- There seems to be no harm caused to participants in any way due to this study.

- It is possible that individuals and health care sector may benefit from the overall findings of the study. The findings can be used to understand the aetiology and epidemiology of a rare disease like lumbar disc prolapse and can be used to generate new health programs and strengthen already running campaigns.

- Tobacco prevention messages can be delivered to the subjects at the end of the study.

> **Privacy, anonymity and confidentiality**

- All collected data will be de-identified.

- Participants, interviewers, hospitals, staff etc. will be identified by numbers and not by personal information.

> **Right not to participate or withdraw**

- All the participants will have an opportunity and right to withdraw from the study at anytime and for any reason, without any prejudice.

7. Discussion and conclusions

There is a need for new research to accurately estimate the incidence and prevalence of lumbar disc prolapse and its association with smoking. The on-going disease burden of lumbar disc prolapse and its most common symptom, back pain, demands that new prevention and management strategies be developed, but these cannot be realised before the aetiology and epidemiology of the disease is understood.

A case-control study is the best study design to achieve this aim. This report presents a protocol for a case-control study across Australia, which appears practically challenging, but seems achievable. Choosing a case-control study design over cohort study design makes it not only cost-efficient but less time-consuming as well.

The strengths of the proposed study include the clarity of the research question, the robustness of the design, the relatively simple statistical analysis and its convenient ethical issues.

Limitations of the study include introduction of selection bias by apparent low response rates among neighbourhood controls. Recall bias, which is common in case-control studies, can be introduced with respect to crucial exposure questions amongst cases. There is also a potential for confounding by unmeasured factors that can lead to bias in the study.

Selecting cases from hospitals across Australia and controls from the neighbourhood of the cases will not only increase response rate but will minimise selection bias as well. Collection of data by trained interviewers through face-to face interviews is not only cost effective but will minimise recall bias and will increase internal validity of the study. It is known that "when self-reported data are used, interviews are probably preferable to self-administered questionnaires as the identity of the responder can be verified, and the use of trained interviewers ensures that participants understand the

questions" (Jan Hartvigsen, Christensen et al. 2004).

Finally, an additional advantage of using case-control study is the potential to

examine multiple exposure factors thereby contributing further to the understanding

of the aetiology and epidemiology of a rare disease like lumbar disc prolapse.

8. References

Afifi, N. M. and K. A. Hafez (2007). "An Experimental Study of the Effects of Nicotine on the Intervertebral Disc." The Egyptian Journal of Hospital Medicine **27**: 128-142.

AIHW (2006). Artificial intervertebral disc replacement (Total disc arthroplasty).

Akmal, M., A. Kesani, et al. (2004). "Effect of nicotine on spinal disc cells: a cellular mechanism for disc degeneration." Spine **29**(5): 568.

Ashton, I., B. Ashton, et al. (1992). "Morphological basis for back pain: the demonstration of nerve fibers and neuropeptides in the lumbar facet joint capsule but not in ligamentum flavum." Journal of Orthopaedic Research **10**(1): 72-78.

Bengtsson, B. and J. Thorson (1991). "Back pain: a study of twins." Acta geneticae medicae et gemellologiae **40**(1): 83.

Braun, W. (1969). Ursachen des lumbalen Bandscheibenvorfalls, Hippokrates-Verlag.

Broetz, D., U. Hahn, et al. (2008). "Lumbar disk prolapse: response to mechanical physiotherapy in the absence of changes in magnetic resonance imaging. Report of 11 cases." Neurorehabilitation **23**(3): 289-294.

Bush, K., N. Cowan, et al. (1992). "The natural history of sciatica associated with disc pathology. A prospective study with clinical and independent radiologic follow-up." Spine **17**(10): 1205.

Cassinelli, E. H. and J. D. Kang (2000). "Current understanding of lumbar disc degeneration." Operative Techniques in Orthopaedics **10**(4): 254-262.

Deyo, R. A., J. D. Loeser, et al. (1990). "Herniated lumbar intervertebral disk." Annals of internal medicine **112**(8): 598-603.

Elwood, J. M. (2007). Critical appraisal of epidemiological studies and clinical trials, Oxford University Press, USA.

Ernst, E. (1993). "Smoking, a cause of back trouble?" Rheumatology **32**(3): 239-242.

Frymoyer, J., M. Pope, et al. (1983). "Risk factors in low-back pain. An epidemiological survey." The Journal of bone and joint surgery. American volume **65**(2): 213-218.

Research project Epidemiology/Biostatistics POPH90219

Grimes, D. A. and K. F. Schulz (2005). "Compared to what? Finding controls for case-control studies." The Lancet 365(9468): 1429-1433.

Gullihorn, L., R. Karpman, et al. (2005). "Differential effects of nicotine and smoke condensate on bone cell metabolic activity." Journal of orthopaedic trauma 19(1): 17.

Heliovaara, M. (1987). "Occupation and risk of herniated lumbar intervertebral disc or sciatica leading to hospitalization." Journal of chronic diseases 40(3): 259-264.

Heliovaara, M., O. Impivaara, et al. (1987). "Lumbar disc syndrome in Finland." Journal of epidemiology and community health 41(3): 251-258.

Heliovaara, M., P. Knekt, et al. (1987). "Incidence and risk factors of herniated lumbar intervertebral disc or sciatica leading to hospitalization." Journal of chronic diseases 40(3): 251-258.

Heliovaara, M., M. Makela, et al. (1991). "Determinants of sciatica and low-back pain." Spine 16(6): 608.

Hestbaek, L., C. Leboeuf-Yde, et al. (2004). "Comorbidity with low back pain: a cross-sectional population-based survey of 12-to 22-year-olds." Spine 29(13): 1483.

Hofmann, F., U. Bolm-Audorff, et al. (1997). "[Occupational diseases of the spine in health care professions--epidemiologic and insurance aspects (I). 1. Review of internationally publicized studies]." Versicherungsmedizin/herausgegeben von Verband der Lebensversicherungs-Unternehmen eV und Verband der Privaten Krankenversicherung eV 49(6): 220.

Hollinger, J. O., J. M. Schmitt, et al. (1999). "Impact of nicotine on bone healing." Journal of biomedical materials research 45(4): 294-301.

Holm, S. and A. Nachemson (1988). "Nutrition of the intervertebral disc: acute effects of cigarette smoking: an experimental animal study." Upsala journal of medical sciences 93(1): 91-99.

Hootman, J., C. Helmick, et al. (2003). "Public health and aging: projected prevalence of self-reported arthritis or chronic joint symptoms among persons aged> 65 years, United States, 2005." MMWR Morb Mortal Wkly Rep 52: 489-491.

Jackson, H. C., R. Winkelmann, et al. (1966). "Nerve endings in the human lumbar spinal column and related structures." The Journal of Bone and Joint Surgery (American) 48(7): 1272-1281.

Jan Hartvigsen, D., K. Christensen, et al. (2004). "Genetic and Environmental Contributions to Back Pain in Old Age." Spine 29(8): 897-902.

Kelsey, J. L. (1975). "An epidemiological study of acute herniated lumbar intervertebral discs." Rheumatology 14(3): 144-159.

Kelsey, J. L., P. B. Githens, et al. (1984). "Acute prolapsed lumbar intervertebral disc. An epidemiologic study with special reference to driving automobiles and cigarette smoking." Spine 9(6): 608.

Kelsey, J. L., P. B. Githens, et al. (1984). "An epidemiologic study of lifting and twisting on the job and risk for acute prolapsed lumbar intervertebral disc." Journal of Orthopaedic Research 2(1): 61-66.

Khan, M., D. Provenza, et al. (1981). "Nicotine toxicity in chick vertebral chondrocytes in vitro." Chem Biol Interact 35: 363-367.

Kirkwood, B. and J. Stern (2003). "Comparing two proportions." Essential medical statistics 2: 148-164.

Komori, H., A. Okawa, et al. (1998). "Contrast-enhanced magnetic resonance imaging in conservative management of lumbar disc herniation." Spine 23(1): 67.

Lawrence, J., M. Molyneux, et al. (1966). "Rheumatism in foundry workers." British journal of industrial medicine 23(1): 42-52.

Liuke, M., S. Solovieva, et al. (2005). "Disc degeneration of the lumbar spine in relation to overweight." International journal of obesity 29(8): 903-908.

Manek, N. J. and A. J. MacGregor (2005). "Epidemiology of back disorders: prevalence, risk factors, and prognosis." Current opinion in rheumatology 17(2): 134-140.

Masui, T., Y. Yukawa, et al. (2005). "Natural history of patients with lumbar disc herniation observed by magnetic resonance imaging for minimum 7 years." Journal of spinal disorders & techniques 18(2): 121.

Mathers, C. D., E. T. Vos, et al. (2001). "The burden of disease and injury in Australia." BULLETIN-WORLD HEALTH ORGANIZATION 79(11): 1076-1084.

Miller, V. M., W. D. Clouse, et al. (2000). "Time and dose effect of transdermal nicotine on endothelial function." American Journal of Physiology-Heart and Circulatory Physiology 279(4): H1913-H1921.

Nachemson, A. (1979). "A critical look at the treatment for low back pain." Scandinavian journal of rehabilitation medicine 11(4): 143.

Ostrum, B. J., M. Romy, et al. (1993). Pathophysiological Basis of lumbar disc degeneration: Imaging analysis, Elsevier.

Pope, M. H., M. Magnusson, et al. (1998). "Low back pain and whole body vibration." Clinical orthopaedics and related research 354: 241.

Powell, M., P. Szypryt, et al. (1986). "Prevalence of lumbar disc degeneration observed by magnetic resonance in symptomless women." The Lancet 328(8520): 1366-1367.

Riihimaki, H. (1991). "Low-back pain, its origin and risk indicators." Scandinavian Journal of Work, Environment & Health 17(2): 81-90.

Rothman, K. J., S. Greenland, et al. (2008). Modern epidemiology, Lippincott Williams & Wilkins.

Scollo, M., M. Winstanley, et al. (2008). Tobacco in Australia: Facts & Issues: a Comprehensive Online Resource, Cancer Council Victoria.

Seidler, A., U. Bolm-Audorff, et al. (2003). "Occupational risk factors for symptomatic lumbar disc herniation; a case-control study." Occupational and environmental medicine 60(11): 821-830.

Silcox III, D. H., S. D. Boden, et al. (1998). "Reversing the inhibitory effect of nicotine on spinal fusion using an osteoinductive protein extract." Spine 23(3): 291.

Trout, J. J., J. A. Buckwalter, et al. (1982). "Ultrastructure of the human intervertebral disc: II. Cells of the nucleus pulposus." The Anatomical Record 204(4): 307-314.

Webb, P. and C. Bain (2011). Essential epidemiology: an introduction for students and health professionals, Cambridge Univ Pr.

Weber, H. (1994). "The natural history of disc herniation and the influence of intervention." Spine 19(19): 2234.

YOUR KNOWLEDGE HAS VALUE

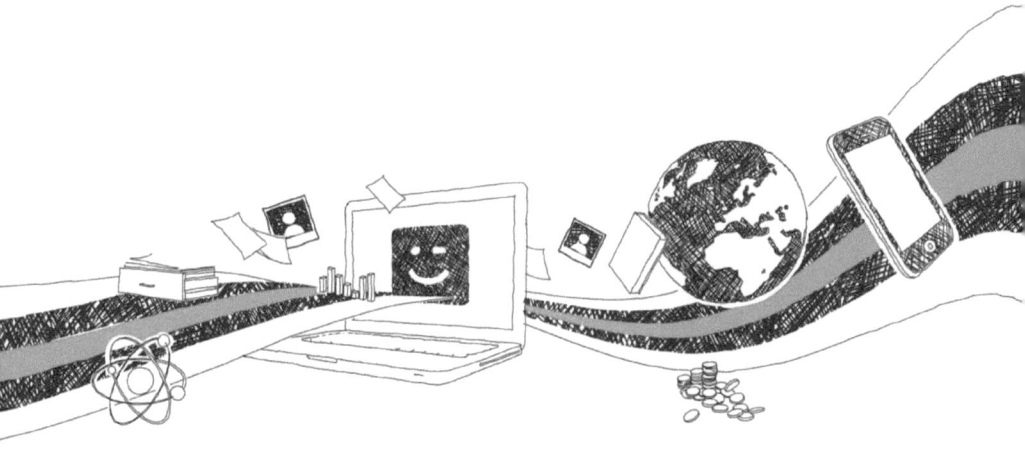

- We will publish your bachelor's and
  master's thesis, essays and papers

- Your own eBook and book -
  sold worldwide in all relevant shops

- Earn money with each sale

Upload your text at www.GRIN.com
and publish for free

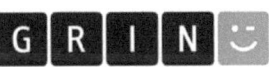